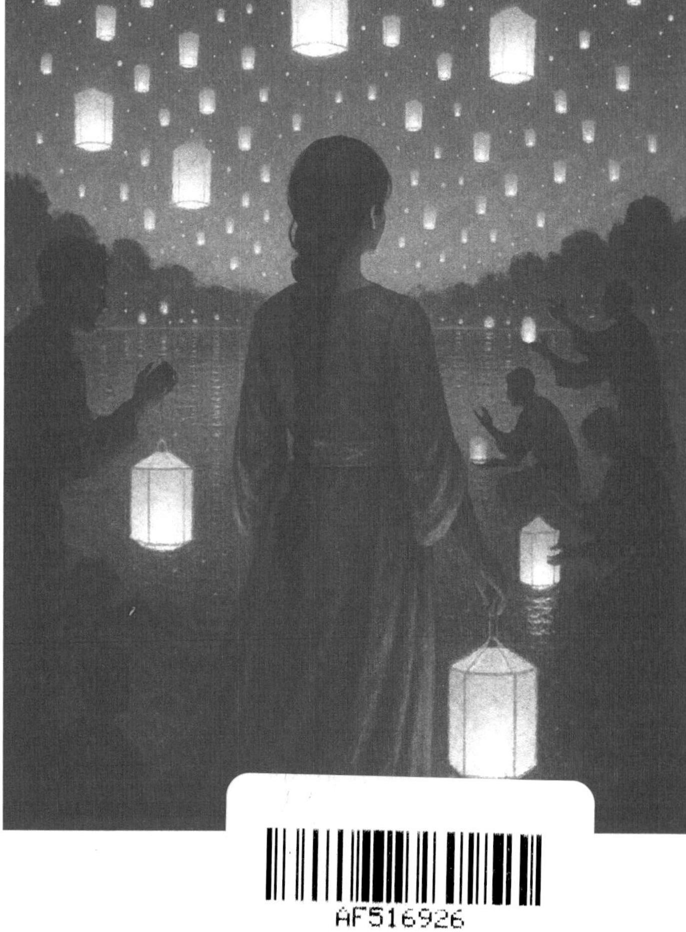

First Published by Ink Gladiators Press®

Translations Of Hope

Editor-in-Chief: Reena Doss

First Edition
ISBN 13: 978-93-49117-29-7

Deep Symbols For You - Lantern 2

Credits:
Book Design by Leonie Belle Hawk
Italian & Arabic Translations: Edited and Proofed
by Justin Adam Wolf and Aelius Arche

Ink Gladiators Press®
Publishing and promoting warriors on life's battlefield
Founded in 2019 | Bangalore, India
www.inkgladiatorspress.com

Love Adores
Never-ending Tales:
Eagerly Ready, News Sails

These main content is written in English,
with Italian and Arabic translations
added after each piece.

To my beloved Weaver,

who is the greatest symbol creator of all things
and who speaks to us in our personal love languages;
this is my awestruck praise to you for giving my mind
a hurricane of layers to uncover your treasures

To my future family,

I think about you with a softness, joy, and care
that the Weaver alone understands;
may we leave behind symbols of our love
full of our mischief wherever we go

To my dear Papa,

who used his playful creativity to make us laugh,
wild games and made-up stories woven into memories;
may the forgotten parts that weren't seen be found
so you realize you left seeds you didn't know you had

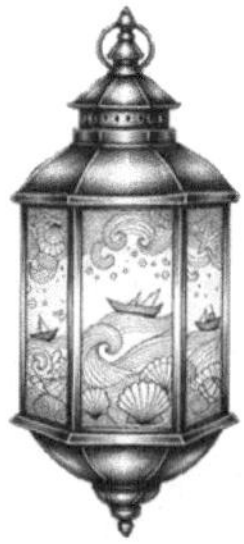

This book is a lantern of

Deep Symbols For You

DEEP SYMBOLS FOR YOU

Because Mental Health Matters

I stopped numbering my pages because my story is still being written.

Besides, I do like its symbol a lot—a sleeping 8.

I'll find you in the dark because I'm the girl

who loves to stay *lost* amongst the midnight stars

caught up with moonbeams *in a lantern*

trying to find my way back *home*

LANTERNS

The pleasure of watching light move across the night sky against its deep purples, blues and greys is an incredible sight to behold.

Though I have never seen it in person myself except on TV, reels or videos, I would imagine that it mimics the feeling of a thousand golden suns glimmering brighter than the stars behind them. I would imagine that it would capture the feeling of remembering that we are each important because no matter how small or big we are light travels faster than sound. I would imagine it would make anyone who sees them smile, open their hearts as hope flutters like birdsong near their door, and the taste of something indescribably good wraps them warmly.

Lanterns are necessary because igniting hope is the best cure in support of mental health awareness. Many live in darkness, in a state of feeling disillusioned by those they put their faith in and have forgotten how to see their own hearts through eyes that love, but a lantern is meant for just this purpose—to relight someone's candle with kindness, to hold a hand steadily in their shadows, and to listen gently to the broken pieces in others speaking. Sometimes, the truth is simple.

That delicate point between human nature and the desire to do what is good is where we will meet the Author of Love. Love can only be known from the One who created us and even when people (who follow God) make us feel like He isn't real or there for us, one of the best ways to reconnect with Him directly is to love with all your heart—and to balance it with healthy discernment, boundaries, and truth in situations where your broken parts might want to do, feel or say the exact opposite. *E.g.: Jesus Christ*

It is my joy to let go of this lantern—as all lanterns must be—for others to find because I want to share something beautiful that I gained and that is mine to offer: You are deeply loved by Heavenly Hands that have constructed, created, and command time, space, and distance.

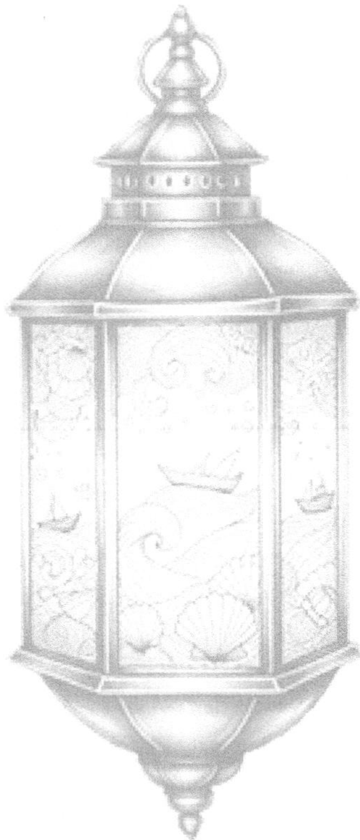

∞

Map

Routes. Trails. Decisions. It is a telescope that frees the wanderer, yet guides a destined path which can be found in a different way. It makes sense of what isn't known, and navigation of them can yield new results when the journey is taken.

I am a thought, a rough outline, a hidden path

Mappa

Percorsi. Sentieri. Decisioni. È il telescopio che libera il vagabondo, ma guida un percorso destinato che può essere trovato in modo diverso. Dà un senso a ciò che non è conosciuto e la navigazione può portare a nuovi risultati quando si intraprende il viaggio.

Sono un pensiero, uno schizzo approssimativo,
un sentiero nascosto

خريطة

طرق. مسارات. قرارات. إنه التلسكوب الذي يحرر المتجول، لكنه يرشد إلى مسار مقدر يمكن العثور عليه بطريقة مختلفة. إنه يفسر ما هو غير معروف، ويمكن أن يؤدي التنقل بينها إلى نتائج جديدة عند القيام بالرحلة.

أنا فكرة، مخطط تقريبي، مسار خفي

Cards

Stories. Games. Connection. They are universally designed—colourful, abstract, and different. Every pack has a wolf with an imprint of standards. Whether it is a spade, a heart, a diamond, a club, a joker, a blank, or a wild card, every single one can break any ice, build fires, boost relationships and bring memories whenever recalled.

I am a thread, a raw filter, a collected pastime

Carte

Storie. Giochi. Connessioni. Sono progettate in modo universale: colorate, astratte e diverse. Ogni mazzo ha un lupo con un'impronta di standard. Che si tratti di un picche, un cuore, un diamante, un fiori, un jolly, una carta bianca o una carta jolly, ognuna di esse può rompere il ghiaccio, accendere fuochi, rafforzare relazioni e riportare alla mente ricordi ogni volta che viene richiamata alla memoria.

Sono un filo conduttore, un filtro grezzo,
un passatempo collezionato

البطاقات

قصص. ألعاب. تواصل. إنها مصممة بشكل عالمي — ملونة، مجردة، ومختلفة. كل حزمة تحتوي على ذئب مع بصمة المعايير. سواء كانت بستوني، قلب، ماسة، نادي، جوكر، بطاقة فارغة، أو بطاقة جامحة، كل واحدة منها يمكنها كسر الجليد، إشعال النيران، تعزيز العلاقات، وجلب الذكريات كلما تم تذكرها.

أنا خيط، مرشح خام، هواية مجمعة

Dictionary

Words. Etymology. Understanding. The power of a word lies in its origin. To use it well is to know its beauty. Not many know this, but every word is a sea, a landscape of cities, worlds and myths hidden under its many layers. Words can hurt those we love, whether intentionally or unintentionally. We must give words to others in the way we want them returned to us.

I am a jewel, a love language, a steady beam

Dizionario

Parole. Etimologia. Comprensione. Il potere di una parola risiede nella sua origine. Usarla bene significa conoscerne la bellezza. Non molti lo sanno, ma ogni parola è un mare, un paesaggio di città, mondi e miti nascosti sotto i suoi numerosi strati. Le parole possono ferire coloro che amiamo, intenzionalmente o meno. Dobbiamo rivolgere agli altri le parole che vorremmo ricevere in cambio.

Sono un gioiello, un linguaggio d'amore, un raggio costante

القاموس

الكلمات. أصل الكلمات. الفهم. تكمن قوة الكلمة في أصلها. لاستخدامها بشكل جيد، يجب معرفة جمالها. لا يعرف الكثيرون ذلك، ولكن كل كلمة هي بحر، ومشهد من المدن والعوالم والأساطير المخبأة تحت طبقاتها العديدة. يمكن للكلمات أن تؤذي من نحبهم، سواء عن قصد أو عن غير .قصد. يجب أن نوجه الكلمات للآخرين بالطريقة التي نريد أن يردوها إلينا

أنا جوهرة، لغة حب، شعاع ثابت

Horse

Wise. Wind. Water. Sunbathers of the land. Dust kickers of the beach. Tender hearts in the world of humanity. They prefer to race in directions with instinct as their compass, rather than guided instruction. They belong to the justice system because they read nature like a blueprint, see the finest truth in energy, and know first-hand what it's like to be freedom without chains.

I am a movie, a wild spirit, a cannon shot

Cavallo

Saggio. Vento. Acqua. Amanti del sole della terra. Calpestatori di polvere della spiaggia. Cuori teneri nel mondo dell'umanità. Preferiscono correre seguendo il loro istinto come bussola, piuttosto che istruzioni guidate. Appartengono al sistema della giustizia perché leggono la natura come un progetto, vedono la verità più profonda nell'energia e conoscono in prima persona cosa significa essere liberi senza catene.

Sono un film, uno spirito selvaggio, un colpo di cannone

الحصان

الحكمة. الريح. الماء. مستمتعو أشعة الشمس على الأرض. مثيرو الغبار على الشاطئ. القلوب .الرقيقة في عالم البشرية. يفضلون الركض في اتجاهات يحددها غريزتهم بدلاً من التعليمات الموجهة ،ينتمون إلى نظام العدالة لأنهم يقرؤون الطبيعة كخريطة، ويرون الحقيقة الأسمى في الطاقة .ويعرفون عن كثب معنى الحرية دون قيود

أنا فيلم، روح جامحة، طلقة مدفع

Calendar

Dates. Months. Years. The realms of a calendar are vast. They can be hung on walls, rest on desks, and be woven into diaries. Why do we want to remember? Because good days are often forgotten when we have a bad day. Because failures are celebratory days. Because the small wins add up to a big one. Because we are glad some people exist, even the ones who made us learn, grow and choose love, rather than be like them. Perhaps it can be used to write favourite lyrics down and create an ingenious table of contents like my father has in his.

I am a scheduler, a rough outline, a hidden path

Calendario

Date. Mesi. Anni. Il mondo dei calendari è vastissimo. Possono essere appesi alle pareti, appoggiati sulle scrivanie e inseriti nei diari. Perché vogliamo ricordare? Perché spesso i giorni belli vengono dimenticati quando ne abbiamo uno brutto. Perché i fallimenti sono giorni da festeggiare. Perché le piccole vittorie si sommano fino a diventare grandi. Perché siamo felici che alcune persone esistano, anche quelle che ci hanno fatto imparare, crescere e scegliere l'amore, piuttosto che essere come loro. Forse può essere usato per scrivere i testi delle canzoni preferite e creare un ingegnoso indice come quello che ha mio padre nel suo.

Sono un pianificatore, uno schizzo approssimativo,

un percorso nascosto

التقويم

التواريخ. الأشهر. السنوات. مجالات التقويم واسعة. يمكن تعليقها على الجدران، ووضعها على المكاتب، ودمجها في اليوميات. لماذا نريد أن نتذكر؟ لأن الأيام الجيدة غالبًا ما تنسى عندما نمر .بأيام سيئة. لأن الفشل هو يوم للاحتفال. لأن الانتصارات الصغيرة تتراكم لتصبح انتصارًا كبيرًا لأننا سعداء بوجود بعض الأشخاص، حتى أولئك الذين جعلونا نتعلم وننمو ونختار الحب، بدلاً من أن نكون مثلهم. ربما يمكن استخدامه لكتابة كلمات الأغاني المفضلة وإنشاء جدول محتويات .مبتكر مثل الذي لدى والدي

أنا مخطط، مخطط تقريبي، مسار خفي

Names

Significance. Holders. Seers. Journeys untold. Whether new or old, simple or complex, deep seas flow within and out. Some names are light, others are shadows. Each syllable is stream carrying memories, twists and dreams of is and what will be. Each name is part of one great destiny—to speak it is to know, to love, to believe that we are already free.

I am a river, a unique sequence, a hidden path

Nomi

Significato. Detentori. Veggenti. Viaggi inconfessabili. Nuovi o antichi, semplici o complessi, mari profondi scorrono dentro e fuori. Alcuni nomi sono luce, altri sono ombre. Ogni sillaba è un flusso che trasporta ricordi, colpi di scena e sogni di ciò che è e di ciò che sarà. Ogni nome fa parte di un unico grande destino: pronunciarlo significa conoscere, amare, credere che siamo già liberi.

Sono un fiume, una sequenza unica, un sentiero nascosto

الأسماء

الأهمية. أصحابها. العرافون. رحلات لم تُروى. سواء كانت جديدة أو قديمة، بسيطة أو معقدة، تتدفق البحار العميقة من الداخل إلى الخارج. بعض الأسماء خفيفة، وبعضها ظلال. كل مقطع لفظي هو تيار يحمل الذكريات والتقلبات والأحلام لما هو موجود وما سيكون. كل اسم هو جزء من مصير عظيم واحد — نطقه يعني المعرفة والحب والإيمان بأننا أحرار بالفعل.

أنا نهر، تسلسل فريد، طريق خفي

Motorcycle

Transformer. Machine. Explorer. Its thunderous roars when the engine starts. There is beast that comes alive when a rider mounts to set out on the open road. It is the motion of feeling your hair escape the helmet to dance in the breeze. It is chasing horizons where the sun meets a new day or kisses the end of it. When life unfolds, and the city fades, new frontiers can never be unnamed.

I am a ride, a windswept machine, a wheeled house

Motocicletta

Trasformatore. Macchina. Esploratore. Il rombo fragoroso quando il motore si avvia. C'è una bestia che prende vita quando un motociclista sale in sella per lanciarsi sulla strada aperta. È la sensazione dei capelli che sfuggono dal casco per danzare nella brezza. È inseguire orizzonti dove il sole incontra un nuovo giorno o ne bacia la fine. Quando la vita si dispiega e la città svanisce, nuove frontiere non possono mai rimanere senza nome.

Sono un viaggio, una macchina spazzata dal vento,
una casa su ruote.

دراجة نارية

محول. آلة. مستكشف. صوت هديرها المدوي عند تشغيل المحرك. هناك وحش يحيي عندما يركب السائق ليخرج إلى الطريق المفتوح. إنها حركة الشعور بشعرك يتحرر من الخوذة ليرقص في النسيم. إنها مطاردة الآفاق حيث تلتقي الشمس بيوم جديد أو تقبل نهايته. عندما تتكشف .الحياة، وتختفي المدينة، لا يمكن أبدًا عدم تسمية الحدود الجديدة

أنا رحلة، آلة تهب عليها الرياح، منزل على عجلات

Art

Questions. Answers. Seeker. A splash of colour and a thought is born. Another colour and the mind escapes the notion of time. Each curve is like find the moon, or its crescent. Each tone, shade and hue is like painting the rays of the sun. Art is truth in fragments, a place where the wild soul can just be—untamed, yet sung and felt deeply in its need.

I am a scribble, a happy unknown, an untamed line

Arte

Domande. Risposte. Ricerca. Uno spruzzo di colore e nasce un pensiero. Un altro colore e la mente sfugge alla nozione di tempo. Ogni curva è come trovare la luna, o la sua falce. Ogni tono, sfumatura e tonalità è come dipingere i raggi del sole. L'arte è verità in frammenti, un luogo dove l'anima selvaggia può semplicemente essere: indomita, ma cantata e sentita profondamente nel suo bisogno.

Sono uno scarabocchio, un felice sconosciuto,
una linea indomita

الفن

.أسئلة. إجابات. باحث. رشة من اللون وتولد فكرة. لون آخر والعقل يهرب من مفهوم الزمن .كل منحنى يشبه العثور على القمر أو هلاله. كل نغمة وظل ولون يشبه رسم أشعة الشمس الفن هو الحقيقة في شظايا، مكان يمكن أن تكون فيه الروح الجامحة على طبيعتها - جامحة، لكنها .تُغنى وتُحس بعمق في حاجتها

.أنا خربشة، مجهول سعيد، خط جامح

Music

Arrows. Meditation. Reflections. It wakes our soul, caress our skin beneath and helps us feel every single thing. It stirs the spirit where numbness aches in days, decades and dreams. It opens our hearts to spill the depths of ink. And when all is lost, and no sound can be heard, there is voice that beats in rhythm—it is the rhythm of the heart.

I am a note, a sweet balm, a loving ache

Musica

Frecce. Meditazione. Riflessioni. Risveglia la nostra anima, accarezza la nostra pelle e ci aiuta a sentire ogni singola cosa. Risveglia lo spirito dove il torpore fa male nei giorni, nei decenni e nei sogni. Apre i nostri cuori per riversarne le profondità. E quando tutto è perduto e non si sente alcun suono, c'è una voce che batte a ritmo: è il ritmo del cuore.

Sono una nota, un dolce balsamo, un dolore amorevole

الموسيقى

الأسهم. التأمل. التأملات. إنها توقظ أرواحنا، وتداعب بشرتنا وتساعدنا على الشعور بكل شيء. إنها تثير الروح حيث يؤلمها الخدر في الأيام والعقود والأحلام. إنها تفتح قلوبنا لتسكب أعماق الحبر. وعندما نفقد كل شيء، ولا نسمع أي صوت، هناك صوت ينبض بإيقاع - إنه إيقاع القلب.

أنا نوتة موسيقية، بلسم حلو، ألم محب

Numbers

Factual. Solace. Creative. Zero marks the beginning and the end. They are endless. Neither cold nor warm. Each have meaning, memory and moments named after them. Some numbers holds pain, creativity and forgiveness. Others are a distant bond that blurs each year. Rare are the ones with mysteries like infinity, and the foot that carries its destiny.

I am a science, a known symmetry, a gentle pattern

Numeri

Reali. Confortanti. Creativi. Lo zero segna l'inizio e la fine. Sono infiniti. Né freddi né caldi. Ognuno ha un significato, un ricordo e momenti a cui prende il nome. Alcuni numeri racchiudono dolore, creatività e perdono. Altri sono un legame lontano che si offusca ogni anno che passa. Rari sono quelli che racchiudono misteri come l'infinito e il piede che ne porta il destino.

Sono una scienza, una simmetria nota, un motivo delicato

الأرقام

واقعية. مريحة. إبداعية. الصفر يمثل البداية والنهاية. إنها لا نهاية لها. ليست باردة ولا دافئة. لكل منها معنى وذاكرة ولحظات سميت باسمها. بعض الأرقام تحمل الألم والإبداع والمغفرة. والبعض الآخر يمثل رابطة بعيدة تتلاشى مع مرور كل عام. نادرة هي الأرقام التي تحمل أسرارًا مثل اللانهاية، والقدم التي تحمل مصيرها.

أنا علم، تناسق معروف، نمط لطيف

Birds

Wings. Weather. Willpower. They are feathers that have brushed with the clouds. They witnessed the piles of humanity's dreams being birthed. Their shapes are crowned with freedom's courage that no cage can ever know. Chains try to catch them, but even when they are hunted, caught, and held, their voices don't stop singing of the sky.

I am a season, a free song, a joyful rhythm

Uccelli

Ali. Tempo atmosferico. Forza di volontà. Sono piume che hanno sfiorato le nuvole. Hanno assistito alla nascita dei sogni dell'umanità. Le loro forme sono coronate dal coraggio della libertà che nessuna gabbia potrà mai conoscere. Le catene cercano di catturarli, ma anche quando vengono cacciati, catturati e imprigionati, le loro voci non smettono di cantare il cielo.

Sono una stagione, una canzone libera, un ritmo gioioso

الطيور

أجنحة. طقس. إرادة. إنها ريشات لمست السحاب. لقد شاهدت أكوام أحلام البشرية وهي تولد. تتوج أشكالها بشجاعة الحرية التي لا يمكن لأي قفص أن يعرفها. تحاول السلاسل الإمساك بها، ولكن حتى عندما يتم اصطيادها والقبض عليها واحتجازها، لا تتوقف أصواتها عن الغناء في السماء.

أنا موسم، أغنية حرة، إيقاع مبهج

Tea

Aromatic. Fragnant. Nourishing. It is a golden moment to sit with a cup of tea, sip its edge in silence, and watch as the steam lifts, dances a bit before chasing the wind to disappear. It is a delight to feel the warmth enter your body and know the noise within grows still. With every refill, peace moves in waves. It is a reminder to take everything in and just be...simply with the tea.

I am a distraction, a small fable, a heated truth

Tè

Aromatico. Profumato. Nutriente. È un momento magico sedersi con una tazza di tè, sorseggiarlo in silenzio e guardare il vapore che sale, danza un po' prima di essere portato via dal vento e scomparire. È una delizia sentire il calore entrare nel corpo e sentire il rumore interiore che si placa. Ad ogni sorso, la pace si diffonde a ondate. È un invito ad accogliere tutto e semplicemente essere... semplicemente con il tè.

Sono una distrazione, una piccola favola, una verità accesa

الشاي

،عطري. معطر. مغذي. إنها لحظة ذهبية أن تجلس مع كوب من الشاي، وترتشفه في صمت وتشاهد البخار يتصاعد، ويرقص قليلاً قبل أن يطارد الريح ليختفي. إنه لمن دواعي السرور أن تشعر بالدفء يدخل جسدك وتدرك أن الضجيج بداخلك يهدأ. مع كل كوب جديد، ينتشر السلام على شكل موجات. إنه تذكير بأن تستوعب كل شيء وتكون على طبيعتك... ببساطة .مع الشاي

أنا إلهاء، حكاية صغيرة، حقيقة ساخنة

Glasses

Clever. Vision. Protection. Don't they seem like windows to see people, the environment and things like as though they were separate worlds? They help eyes correct sight to the best of their capacity for the most part. But I have often found them to be the perfect escape to be absent from reality. Not many pay attention to the ones in glasses. It is like having an invisibility cloak that sees truth without the fog of others' perceptions.

I am a researcher, a black frame, a loud observer

Occhiali

Intelligenti. Visione. Protezione. Non sembrano finestre attraverso cui vedere le persone, l'ambiente e le cose come se fossero mondi separati? Aiutano gli occhi a correggere la vista al meglio delle loro capacità, per la maggior parte. Ma spesso li ho trovati il rifugio perfetto per assentarmi dalla realtà. Non molti prestano attenzione a chi porta gli occhiali. È come avere un mantello dell'invisibilità che permette di vedere la verità senza la nebbia delle percezioni altrui.

Sono un ricercatore, una montatura nera,

un osservatore rumoroso

النظارات

ذكية. رؤية. حماية. ألا تبدو وكأنها نوافذ نرى من خلالها الناس والبيئة والأشياء كما لو كانت .عوالم منفصلة؟ إنها تساعد العينين على تصحيح الرؤية إلى أقصى حد ممكن في معظم الأحيان لكنني غالبًا ما أجدها الملاذ المثالي للهروب من الواقع. لا ينتبه الكثيرون إلى من يرتدون .النظارات. إنها مثل عباءة خفية ترى الحقيقة دون ضباب تصورات الآخرين

.أنا باحث، إطار أسود، مراقب صاخب

Deep Symbols For You

Space For You

Reena Doss

Acknowledgements

I am grateful

Symbols have always held a lasting, sentimental value in my understanding of events, people, and life itself. I am always careful to research the deep layers of every symbol. I do not take risks with symbolism that has no root in my own history. This is because the grace that covered me in the places that brought either joy or sorrow can only be claimed by me—not always through the same wound or path, but through the deeper ones available to us when we meet the One who is already victorious, and whose grace we can claim in confidence.

I want to thank my loved ones for reminding me of the symbols in my life that have meant so much to me. They were seeds that hadn't yet felt ready—until they were. The few symbols in these books were inspired by my father, James Doss, who has always found symbols to hold deeper significance in the grand scheme of things. This is a love language that is unique to each of us and does need to be taught because it is deeply woven into our experiences with those we love, with the events that shaped us, and with the Weaver Himself.

Most importantly, I thank the Weaver for teaching me many love languages—their layers, their symbols, and their wild hearts—every time I reached for Him. I also thank my team at *Ink Gladiators Press—Leonie Belle Hawk, Justin Adam Wolf* and *Aelius Arche* for being my constant companions, for wearing many hats, and for helping me do all the work that I needed to do under different names.

May the quill of hope find you in the dark,

Reena Doss

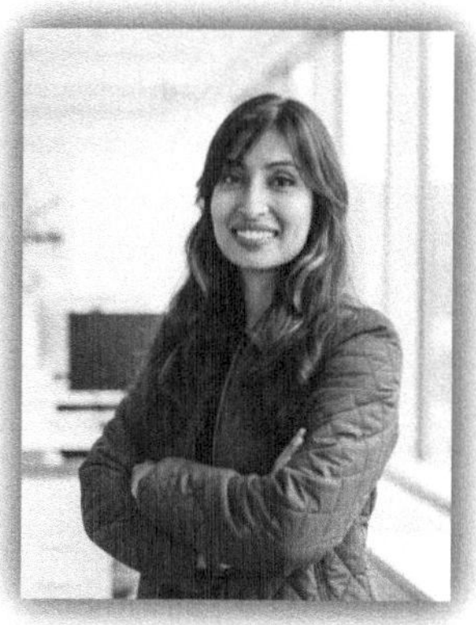

I'll find you in the dark...

Born in Calcutta with roots drawn from Chennai and Pondicherry, Reena Doss has lived most of her life in the south of India—Bangalore. Though she prefers traveling to far-off places inside her head, she sometimes ventures into the world that others call real.

Reena Doss considers writing to be her first voice of expression, followed closely by art, and creativity. Through the encouraging platform provided by the Instagram community, she reclaimed her lost voices, evolved a few others and discovered new ones along the way.

This has redeemed her trust that consistent Hope, Faith and Love in what is true ignites what is impossible to occur. Her adoration for her beloved Weaver, the Celestial Sky, Nature and her fellow Earthians has given her immeasurable courage to endure every season with a resilience born from battles overcome.

You can try and catch her but it may not always be possible as she is generally off on adventures flying on phoenix wings, swimming into the deep with mermaids and chasing fiery dragons down for stories.

To those who remain true to themselves,
to those who create magic wherever they go,
and for those who sit beside the hurt
when everyone else leaves,
Art will always immortalize you.

Please scan the QR code to follow her on
Instagram @reenadossauthor
www.reenadoss.com

This little book is called a *Lantern* because love is light in disguise. It can only be found when you are buried in the dark, when the seeds die, and you choose to bravely grow and become worthy of your given name—a polished gem, a diamond that cannot help but shine. Lanterns are meant for those who need hope while they are being:

- ♥ Condemned unjustly by those who see a version they want
- ♥ Gossiped about when they are not present to defend themselves
- ♥ Taken advantage of when they were beaten down by life, by those who should have stood by them
- ♥ Judged, neglected, and persecuted while they are struggling
- ♥ Abandoned by those who willingly chose to see them as toxic because it suited their narrative
- ♥ Manipulated by those who bore false witness against them to take what wasn't theirs
- ♥ Gaslit, broken, and their truth erased while they were at their most vulnerable
- ♥ Hated, harassed, and purposefully pressured into giving up on who they are because of others' jealousy
- ♥ Trying to process trauma to speak in a language that isn't being heard
- ♥ Eagerly isolated by loved ones on the advice of others who can't understand them any more
- ♥ Neglected by those whose promises dimmed when things got difficult
- ♥ Treated as outcasts by those who expect their will to be done
- ♥ Mocked for what they do just because it is different and does not fit into any box

Promoting hope and unwrapping the stigma of mental health

For any inquiries, please email us at contact@inkgladiatorspress.com.

Please scan the QR Code below if you would like to follow us

on Instagram @inkgladiatorspress.

Ink Gladiators Press®

Publishing and promoting warriors on life's battlefield

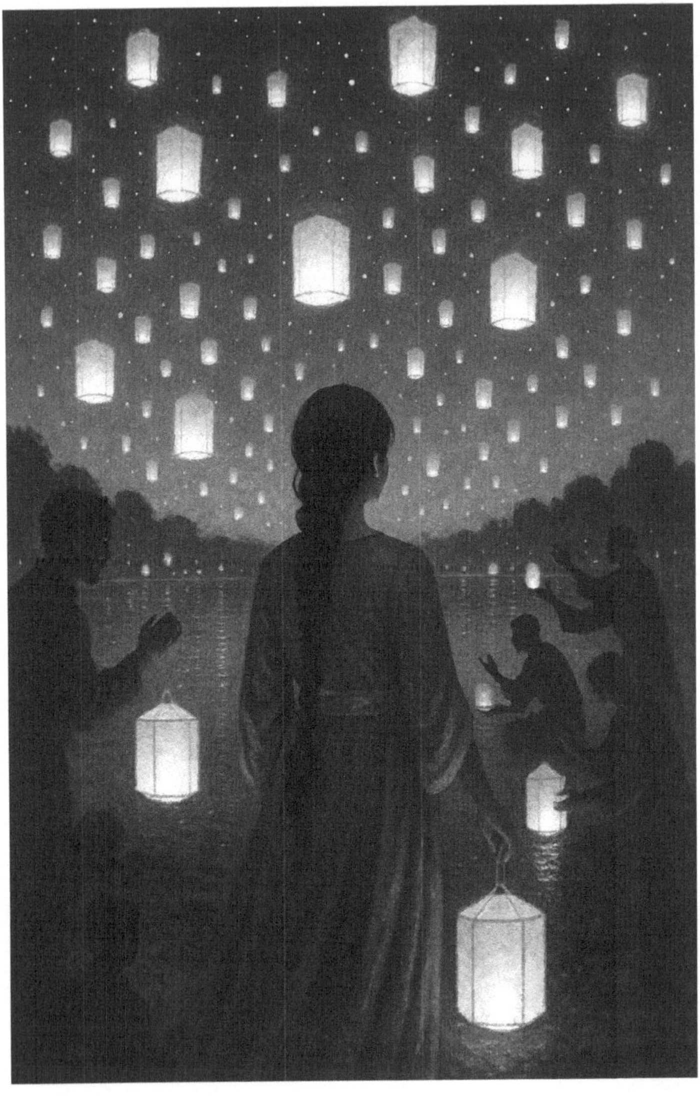

9 789349 117297

Printed at Repro India Ltd.